Keto Slow Cooker Best Recipes

A Handful of 50 Quick, Delicious Recipes for Your Keto Meals

Katherine Lowe

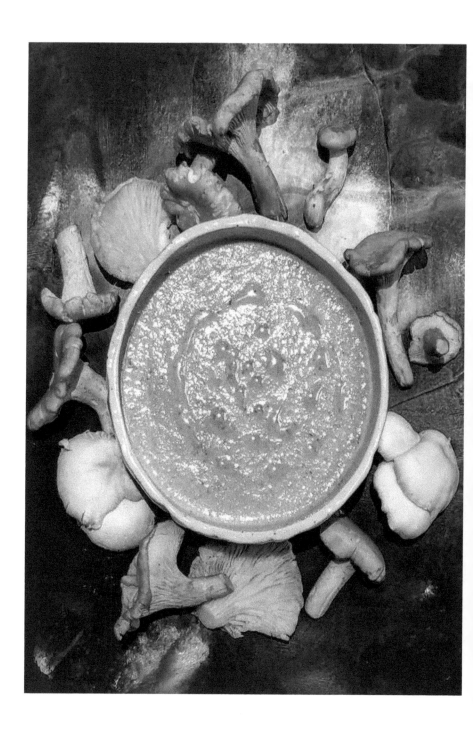

sources. Please consult a licensed professional before attempting any techniques outlined in this book.

By reading this document, the reader agrees that under no circumstances is the author responsible for any losses, direct or indirect, which are incurred as a result of the use of information contained within this document, including, but not limited to, — errors, omissions, or inaccuracies.

Table of Contents

Sticky Sesame Cauliflower Slow Cooker Bites

Preparation time: 15 minutes

Cooking time: 2 hours

Servings: 4

Ingredients:

- 1-pound cauliflower
- ½ teaspoon paprika
- ½ teaspoon ground cumin
- 1 teaspoon garlic powder
- 1 teaspoon sesame oil
- 1/3 cup honey
- 2 tablespoons apple cider vinegar
- 1 teaspoon sweet chili sauce
- 3 garlic cloves, minced
- ¼ cup of water
- 1 tablespoon arrowroot powder or cornstarch
- 1 cup green onions to garnish
- Sesame seeds to garnish

Directions:

1. Place all spices, minus the green onions and sesame seeds, in a bowl, and cover the cauliflower thoroughly with the mixture. Place the cauliflower into the slow cooker.

2. Add the rest of the ingredients and cover. Cook on low for 2 hours. The sauce will thicken with the cornstarch or arrowroot powder. When done, remove each bite and garnish with toasted sesame seeds and green onion slices on top.

Nutrition:

- Calories: 240
- Fat: 7g
- Protein: 3g
- Carbs: 18g

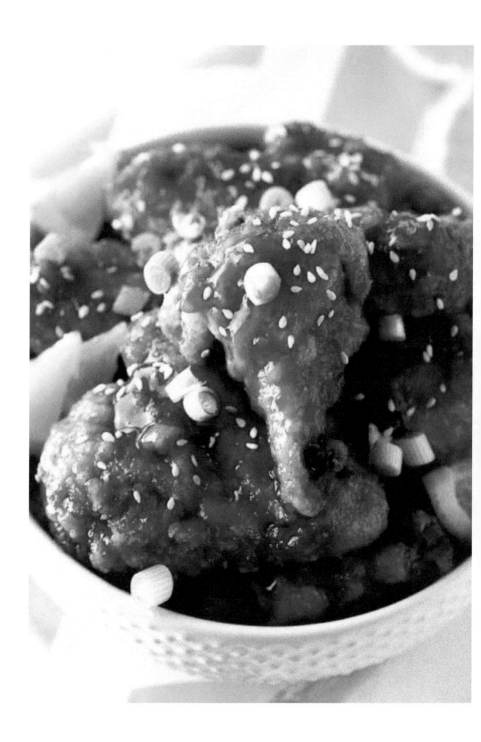

Crockpot Cauliflower Mac and Cheese

Preparation time: 15 minutes

Cooking time: 4 hours

Servings : 4

Ingredients:

- 1-pound cauliflower
- 2 cups shredded cheddar cheese
- 2 ½ cups milk
- 1 12-ounce can evaporate milk
- ½ tablespoon mustard

Directions:

1. Place all of the fixings above in the slow cooker and put on low for 3 hours until most of the liquid has been absorbed.

2. Sprinkle some extra cheese on top and cook for 15 minutes until it has melted and the rest of the liquid is absorbed. Garnish with some parsley and even shredded parmesan cheese.

Nutrition:

- Calories: 215
- Fat: 4g

- Protein: 3g
- Carbs: 18g

Crockpot Vegetable Lasagna

Preparation time: 15 minutes

Cooking time: 2 hours

Servings: 4

Ingredients:

- 2 medium zucchinis
- 1 medium eggplant
- 2 cups tomato-based pasta sauce
- 1 red onion, diced
- 1 red bell pepper, diced
- 16 ounces low fat cottage cheese
- 2 large eggs
- 8 ounces shredded Mozzarella
- 2 tablespoons basil, chopped
- 2 tablespoons parmesan cheese, for garnish

Directions:

1. Slice eggplant plus zucchini lengthwise into thin strips, approximately ¼ inch thick so that they resemble the shape of lasagna noodles. Spread them out over a layer of paper towels and toss with salt.

2. Let stand for 15 minutes to absorb the salt. It helps the vegetables to absorb the liquid. Lightly coat the bottom of your crockpot and spread ½ cup of tomato sauce along the bottom.

3. In a separate bowl, beat the eggs and cottage cheese. Create a layer of "noodles," then 1/3 of the cottage cheese mixture, 1/3 of the bell peppers and onions, and 1/3 of the mozzarella and tomato sauce.

4. Put down another layer of "noodles," then repeat. Finish with the third layer of "noodles." Cook on high for 2 hours, until the eggplant is tender. Slice and scoop out portions as desired, then garnish with herbs and cheese.

Nutrition:

- Calories: 213
- Fat: 9g
- Protein: 3g
- Carbs: 18g

Tasty Tagine Five a Day

Preparation time: 15 minutes

Cooking time: 8 hours

Servings: 6

Ingredients:

- 4 tablespoons of olive oil
- 1 sliced red onion
- 2 cloves of crushed garlic
- 500 grams of aubergine in 1 cm-thick slice, cut lengthways
- 300 grams of quartered ripe tomatoes
- 1 small sliced fennel bulb
- 50 grams of sundried tomatoes
- 1 teaspoon of coriander seeds

For the dressing:

- 100 grams of feta cheese, and extra for topping
- 50 grams of toasted almond flakes

Directions:

1. Put two tbsp of olive oil into the slow cooker and add the crushed garlic and the onions. Brush the aubergines with

the remaining olive oil and place them on top of the onions and garlic.

2. Arrange the sundried tomatoes, fennel slices, and the tomatoes around the aubergines. Flavor it with salt plus pepper and pour the coriander seeds over the top. Cook for 6-8 hours on low.

3. Place the dressing ingredients into a food processor and work until smooth. Spoon the vegetables onto serving dishes, drizzle the dressing over the top and crumble the feta cheese on top.

Nutrition:

- Calories: 289
- Fat: 20g
- Carbs: 11g
- Protein: 8g

Baked Mushrooms with Pesto & Ricotta

Preparation time: 15 minutes

Cooking time: 6 hours

Servings: 4

Ingredients:

- 5 tablespoons of olive oil, extra virgin
- 16 large chestnut mushrooms
- A 250-gram tub of ricotta
- 2 tablespoons of pesto
- 2 finely chopped cloves of garlic
- 25 grams of freshly grated parmesan cheese
- 2 tablespoons of fresh, chopped parsley

Directions:

1. Slice the mushroom stems level with the caps. In a small bowl, combine the garlic, pesto, and ricotta, and spoon into the mushroom heads.

2. Place the mushroom caps in a slow cooker and cook on low for 4-6 hours. In the last half-hour, sprinkle the parmesan cheese over the top of the mushrooms. Serve topped with the fresh parsley.

Nutrition:

- Calories: 400
- Fat: 34g
- Carbohydrates: 2g
- Protein: 19g

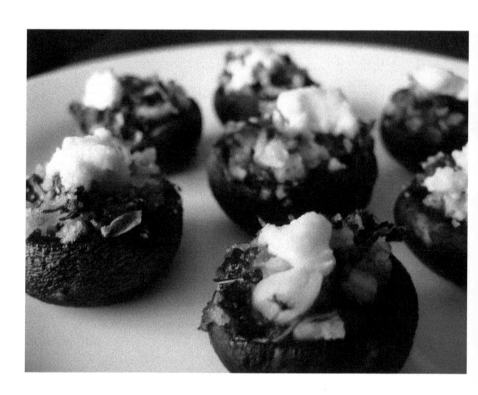

Dal with Crispy Onions

Preparation time: 15 minutes

Cooking time: 6 hours

Servings: 4

Ingredients:

- 250 grams of black urad beans
- 100 grams of ghee or butter
- 2 large onions thinly sliced
- 3 cloves of crushed garlic
- 1 piece of ginger, thumb-sized and finely chopped
- 2 teaspoons of ground cumin
- 2 teaspoons of ground coriander
- 1 teaspoon of ground turmeric
- 1 teaspoon of paprika
- ¼ teaspoon of chili powder
- A small bunch of fresh coriander, reserve the leaves and finely chop the stems
- 400 grams of passata
- 1 red chili, pierced with the tip of a knife
- 50 ml of double cream

For serving:

- Baked sweet potato

- Naan bread
- Cooked rice
- Coriander
- Sliced red chili
- Lime wedges
- Yogurt, cream, or swirl
- Indian chutney or pickle
- Crispy salad onions

Directions:

1. Soak the beans within 4 hours or overnight in cold water. Dissolve the ghee or butter in a large saucepan, then add the ginger, onions, and garlic and cook for 15 minutes to caramelize the onions.

2. Add the coriander stems, spices, and 100ml of water. Pour the ingredients into the slow cooker and add the chili, passata, beans, and 400ml water. Season and cook for 5-6 hours on low.

3. When cooked, the beans should be tender, and the dal should be very thick. Add the cream and serve with a side dish of your choice.

Nutrition:

- Calories: 527
- Fat: 34g

- Carbs: 35g
- Protein: 19g

Warming Bean and Veg Soup

Preparation time: 15 minutes

Cooking time: 8 hours

Servings: 4

Ingredients:

- 2 minced garlic cloves
- 1 medium-sized potato, diced
- 2 carrots, peeled and sliced
- 2 celery stalks, diced
- A handful of frozen broad beans
- 2 tins of butter beans
- Paprika
- Worcestershire sauce
- Chili
- Salt and pepper
- Parmesan cheese
- Fresh herbs of your choice

Directions:

1. Put all the fixing except the Parmesan cheese and the fresh herbs in the slow cooker. Cook on low for 8-10 hours. Spoon onto dishes, top with Parmesan cheese and fresh herbs, and serve.

Nutrition:

- Calories: 527
- Carbohydrates: 5.2g
- Fat: 8g
- Protein: 3.7g
- Fiber: 7.4g

Slow-Cooked Baked Beans

Preparation time: 15 minutes

Cooking time: 8 hours

Servings: 8

Ingredients:

- 1 pound of beans of your choice, dried
- 1 diced medium onion
- 1/3 cup of brown sugar
- 1/3 cup of molasses
- ¼ cup of tomato sauce
- 2 tablespoons of yellow mustard
- 1 tablespoon of smoked paprika
- 1 tablespoon of Worcestershire sauce
- 1 tablespoon of cider vinegar or white balsamic vinegar
- Salt and pepper

Directions:

1. Rinse the dried beans, and pour them into the slow cooker, cover them with 2 inches of water and leave them to soak overnight.

2. The following morning, drain the water from the slow cooker and add the remaining ingredients. Put 2 and ½ cups of water, salt, and pepper to season. Cook for 8 hours on low. Spoon onto dishes and serve.

Nutrition:

- Calories: 136
- Fat: 0.2g
- Carbohydrates: 30.4g
- Protein: 3.8g

Peppers Stuffed with Black Beans & Quinoa

Preparation time: 15 minutes

Cooking time: 6 hours

Servings: 6

Ingredients:

- 6 bell peppers
- 1 cup of uncooked quinoa
- 1 can of black beans, drained
- 1 ½ cups of red enchilada sauce
- 1 teaspoon of cumin
- 1 teaspoon of chili powder
- 1 teaspoon of onion powder
- ½ a teaspoon of garlic salt
- 1 ½ cups of Pepper jack cheese, shredded, divided
- Cilantro
- Avocado
- Sour cream

Directions:

1. Cut the tops off the peppers and scrape out the insides. Combine 1 cup of cheese, spices, enchilada sauce, beans, and quinoa in a large bowl and stir thoroughly.

2. Stuff the mixture into the peppers. Pour ½ cup of water into the slow cooker. Arrange the peppers in the water. Cover and cook on high low for 6 hours.

3. Take the lid off and sprinkle the peppers with the remaining cheese, cover and cook for a few minutes to melt the cheese. Serve with avocado, sour cream, and cilantro.

Nutrition:

- Calories: 116
- Fat: 12.9g
- Carbohydrates: 59.5g
- Protein: 22.7g

Eggplant Parmesan

Preparation time: 15 minutes

Cooking time: 8 hours

Servings: 12

Ingredients:

- 4 pounds of eggplant
- 1 tablespoon of salt
- 3 large eggs
- ¼ cup of milk
- 1 ½ cup of breadcrumbs
- 3 ounces of parmesan cheese
- 2 teaspoons of Italian seasoning
- 4 cups of marinara sauce
- 16 ounces of mozzarella cheese

Directions:

1. Slice the peeled eggplant into 1/3 inch-rounds. Put the eggplant in a colander, then sprinkle each layer with salt. Let sit for 30 minutes and then rinse and pat dry.

2. Spread ½ cup of sauce on the bottom of the slow cooker. In a small bowl, whisk the milk and eggs.

3. In another small bowl, whisk the Italian seasoning, Parmesan cheese, and breadcrumbs. Soak the eggplant into the egg batter and then into the breadcrumb mixture.

4. Layer 1/3 of the slices in the slow cooker. Pour 1 cup of sauce and the mozzarella cheese over the top. Repeat twice, cover, and cook for 8 hours. Divide onto plates and serve.

Nutrition:

- Calories: 258
- Carbohydrates: 23g
- Fat: 6g
- Protein: 16g

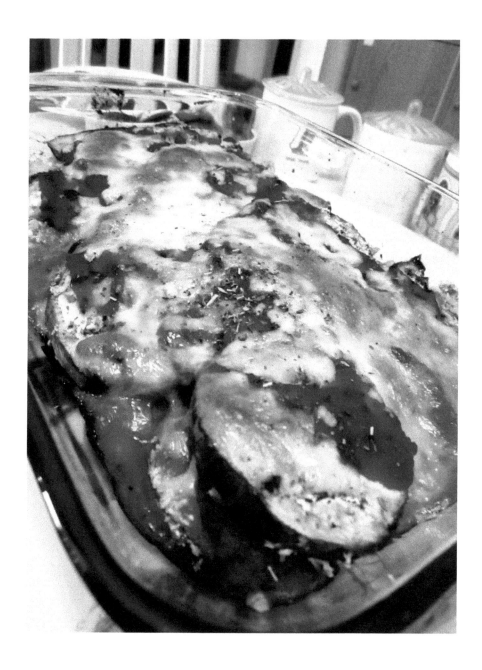

Chili Lentils and Beans

Preparation time: 15 minutes

Cooking time: 8 hours

Servings: 7

Ingredients:

- 1 finely chopped onion
- 3 garlic cloves, minced
- 1 stalk of celery, chopped
- 2 chopped bell peppers
- 1 can of diced tomatoes
- 4 cups of vegetable broth
- 1 can of water
- 1 cup of dried lentils
- 1 can of Bush's Pinto Beans
- 2 tablespoons of chili powder
- 2 teaspoons of cumin
- 1 tablespoon of oregano

Directions:

1. Put all of the fixings into the slow cooker and cook for 8 hours on low. Serve with a combination of cilantro, green onion, avocado, sour cream, plain Greek Yogurt, and shredded cheese.

Nutrition:

- Calories: 192
- Carbs: 25g
- Fat: 2g
- Protein: 13g

Butternut Macaroni Squash

Preparation time: 15 minutes

Cooking time: 8 hours

Servings: 5

Ingredients:

- 1 ½ cups of butternut squash, cubed
- ½ cup of chopped tomatoes
- 1 ½ cups of water
- 2 minced garlic cloves
- A handful of fresh thyme, finely chopped
- A handful of fresh rosemary, finely chopped
- ¼ cup of nutritional yeast
- 1 cup of non-dairy milk
- 1 ½ cups of whole wheat macaroni
- Salt and pepper

Directions:

1. Add the butternut squash, diced tomatoes, water, garlic, thyme, and rosemary to the slow cooker. Cover and cook on low within 7-9 hours.

2. Transfer the ingredients from the slow cooker into a food processor and add the nutritional yeast, half a cup of non-dairy milk, and blend.

3. Pour the ingredients back into the slow cooker, add the macaroni, cover, and cook for a further 20 minutes on high. Stir, cook for a further 25 minutes and add salt and pepper to taste. Spoon onto dishes and serve.

Nutrition:
- Calories: 187
- Fat: 2g
- Carbohydrates: 35g
- Protein: 8g

Veggie Pot Pie

Preparation time: 15 minutes

Cooking time: 4 hours

Servings: 6

Ingredients:

- 6-7 cups of chopped veggies of your choice
- ½ cup of diced onions
- 4 minced garlic cloves
- Fresh thyme, finely chopped
- ½ cup of flour
- 2 cups of chicken broth
- ¼ cup of cornstarch
- ¼ cup of heavy cream
- Salt and pepper
- 1 thawed frozen puff pastry sheet
- 2 tablespoons of butter

Directions:

1. Put the chopped veggies in the slow cooker, put the garlic and onions. Add the flour. Add the broth and stir until everything is well blended. Cover and cook for 3-4 hours on high.

2. In a small bowl, combine the cornstarch and ¼ cup of water and whisk thoroughly. Put the cornstarch mix in the slow cooker.

3. Add the cream, cover, and continue to cook until the mixture thickens approximately 15 minutes. Transfer the vegetable mixture into a baking dish.

4. Lay the puff pastry over the top. Melt the butter and brush it over the top of the pastry. Bake at 350 degrees for 10 minutes until the pastry turns fluffy and golden. Divide onto dishes and serve.

Nutrition:

- Calories: 325
- Fat: 0.8g
- Protein: 4.5g
- Carbohydrates: 6.7g

Barbecue Beef Stew

Preparation time: 15 minutes

Cooking time: 8 hours

Servings: 6

Ingredients:

¾ cup of each:

- Homemade tomato paste
- Balsamic vinegar
- ½ tsp black pepper

1 teaspoon of each:

- Smoked paprika
- Kosher salt
- Garlic powder
- 2 tbsp. sweetener

For the Stew:

- 1 tsp kosher salt
- 2 lb. extra-lean stew beef meat/boneless chuck roast
- 1 tbsp. olive oil
- ½ t. black pepper
- 2 tbsp. cold tap water
- 1 tbsp cornstarch or ½ t. konjac flour

- Also Needed: 14-inch skillet

Directions:

1. Chop the meat into one-inch pieces, and season it with pepper and salt. Combine the barbecue sauce ingredients.

2. Prepare the skillet by adding half of the oil using the med-high setting for three minutes. Add half of the beef and cook for about five minutes.

3. Place in the slow cooker. Add the rest of the oil and cook the second half of beef and add it also. Empty the sauce over the prepared meat and stir. Place the top on the pot and cook for 7 ½ hours on low.

4. Whisk in the cornstarch and water in a dish until smooth. Empty it into the beef juices. Set the slow cooker on high for 30 minutes. When thickened to your liking, serve, and enjoy.

Nutrition:

- Calories: 445
- Carbs: 10g
- Protein: 30g
- Fat: 29g

Beef Stew with Tomatoes

Preparation time: 15 minutes

Cooking time: 8 hours

Servings: 6

Ingredients:

- 1 pkg. (5lbs.) stew beef
- 2 cans chili-ready diced tomatoes (14.5oz.) - organic
- 2 tsp hot sauce
- 1 cup of beef broth
- 1 tbsp. of each:
- Chili mix (pre-packaged)
- Worcestershire sauce
- Salt to taste

Directions:

1. Warm up the slow cooker in the high setting. Add the stewing beef, tomatoes, hot sauce, broth, Worcestershire sauce, chili mix, and salt in the slow cooker.

2. Set the timer for six hours. Break the meat apart and continue cooking for another two hours. Sprinkle with a pinch of salt to taste when ready to serve.

Nutrition:

- Calories: 222
- Carbs: 9g
- Fat: 7g
- Protein: 27g

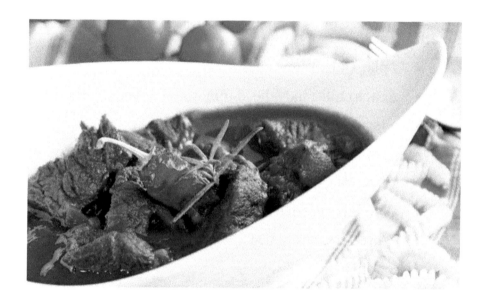

Chicken Stew

Preparation time: 15 minutes

Cooking time: 2 hours

Servings: 4

Ingredients:

- 1 pkg. (28oz.) skinless & deboned chicken thighs
- 2 celery sticks, diced
- ½ cup diced of each:
- Onion
- 2 medium carrots – approx.
- 2 cup of chicken stock
- ½ tsp dried rosemary/1 fresh sprig
- 3 minced garlic cloves
- Pepper and salt to taste
- ½ tsp dried oregano
- ¼ tsp dried thyme
- ½ cup of heavy cream
- 1 cup of fresh spinach
- Xanthan gum as desired (start at 1/8 tsp)
- Recommended: 3-quart or larger slow cooker

Directions:

1. Dice the chicken into one-inch chunks. Remove the skin, and finely dice the carrots and celery. Add the veggies and chicken to the slow cooker.

2. Pour in the stock, thyme, oregano, rosemary, and garlic in the cooker. Toss in the pepper and salt. Mix in the heavy cream and spinach leaves.

3. Add the xanthan gum to thicken the juices, and simmer another ten minutes. Set the cooker on high for two hours or low setting for four hours. When it's done, enjoy.

Nutrition:

- Calories: 228
- Carbs: 6g
- Fat: 11g
- Protein: 23g

Hare Stew

Preparation time: 15 minutes

Cooking time: 5 hours

Servings: 6

Ingredients:

- ½ lb. uncured organic bacon/smoked pork belly
- 1 whole rabbit/hare (3lb.) cut into pieces
- 2 tbsp. butter
- 2 cups of dry white wine
- 1 large of each:
- Sweet onion
- Sprig of rosemary
- 1 tsp whole peppercorn
- 2 bay leaves
- 2 tbsp. Celtic sea salt

Directions:

1. Cut the pork belly into one-inch bites. Place them in a heated skillet along with the butter. Thinly slice the onion, and toss it in.

2. Continue cooking slowly for approximately five minutes and remove the onion (leaving the grease in the skillet).

Arrange the prepared meat bites in the pan, and continue cooking using the high setting until browned.

3. Pour in the wine, then simmer for two more minutes. Add all the fixings into the slow cooker. Shake in the rosemary, salt, bay leaves, and peppercorn. Select the low setting for five hours. When done, serve, and enjoy.

Nutrition:

- Calories: 517
- Protein: 36g
- Carbs: 2g
- Fat: 32

Herb Chicken & Mushroom Stew

Preparation time: 15 minutes

Cooking time: 4 hours

Servings: 5

Ingredients:

- 1lb. raw chicken tenders
- 24oz. whole white button mushrooms

½ tsp dried of each:

- Oregano
- Basil
- 3 garlic cloves
- ¼ tsp dried thyme
- 1 cup of chicken broth
- 2 bay leaves
- Pepper
- Salt
- 2 tbsp. butter
- ¼ cup of heavy whipping cream
- 8 bacon slices – chopped & cooked
- ¼ cup of freshly chopped parsley

Directions:

1. Cut the stems on the larger mushrooms and wash. Dice into bite-sized pieces and place them in the slow cooker.

2. Arrange the chicken in the pot along with the spices (garlic, basil thyme, oregano, and bay leaves) and broth. Give it a shake of the pepper and salt.

3. Set the timer for three to four hours using the low-temperature setting. Combine the butter and whipping cream. Jazz it up with some salt and pepper to your liking. Serve with the parsley and bacon bits.

Nutrition:

- Calories: 297.2
- Carbs: 4.42g
- Fat: 17.5g
- Protein: 29.99g

Hungarian Beef Goulash

Preparation time: 15 minutes

Cooking time: 4 hours

Servings: 8

Ingredients:

- 2 lb. beef stew meat – cubed
- 2 garlic cloves
- 1 cup of onion – chopped
- 1 tsp salt

2 tbsp. of each:

- Hungarian paprika
- Butter/bacon grease
- ½ tsp of each:
- Caraway seeds
- Pepper
- 2 sliced celery stalks
- 1 yellow/green chopped bell pepper
- 2 cup of cubed daikon radishes
- 1 can (15oz.) diced tomatoes
- 1 ½ cup of beef/chicken broth
- 1 bay leaf

Directions:

1. Prepare a skillet with the butter using the medium heat setting until it's melted. Stir in the onions and cook until translucent. Toss in the paprika and garlic, stirring for another minute.

2. Add the beef, and sprinkle with the pepper, salt, and caraway seeds into the cooker. Fold in the peppers, radish, celery, broth, bay leaf, and tomatoes.

3. Mix thoroughly and prepare using the low setting for six hours. You can also choose four hours using the high setting. Serve!

Nutrition:

- Calories: 345
- Carbs: 5.52g
- Fat: 23.88g
- Protein: 23.84g

Vegetable Beef Stew

Preparation time : 15 minutes

Cooking time: 7 hours

Servings: 10

Ingredients :

- 1 lb. boneless beef braising steaks
- 1 ½ tsp salt – ex. pink Himalayan
- Freshly ground black pepper
- ½ cup of tallow/lard/ghee
- 1 medium white onion
- 4 garlic cloves
- 1 cup of vegetable stock/broth/water
- 2 tbsp. ground cumin

1 tsp of each:

- Turmeric powder
- Ground coriander seeds
- Paprika
- Chili powder
- Ground ginger
- 2 cinnamon sticks
- 1 can (14.1oz.) unsweetened tomatoes – chopped
- 4-5 medium zucchini

- 2 bay leaves
- 1 medium rutabaga – 1.3 lb.
- Suggested: 6-quart slow cooker

Directions:

1. Warm up the cooker on the high setting. Dry the liquids off the steaks with a paper towel. Give the meat a shake of the salt and pepper.

2. Sear the steaks in a skillet with ¼ cup of the butter/ghee. Add to the slow cooker. Peel and dice the garlic and onion. Toss it into the pan with the rest of the ghee.

3. Pour in the tomatoes, turmeric, coriander seeds, chili powder, broth, cumin, and paprika. Gently combine and add to the slow cooker on top of the meat.

4. Put the bay leaves and cinnamon sticks in the cooker. Put the top on the pot. Cook for three hours, and then add the rutabaga on the side of the meat.

5. Cook another hour and add the diced zucchini. Mix and remove the cinnamon sticks and bay leaves when done. Cook for two additional hours. If desired, sprinkle with more pepper and salt. Top it off with some of the fresh herbs and enjoy.

Nutrition:

- Calories: 533

- Carbs: 9.1g
- Fat: 39.5g
- Protein: 31.9g

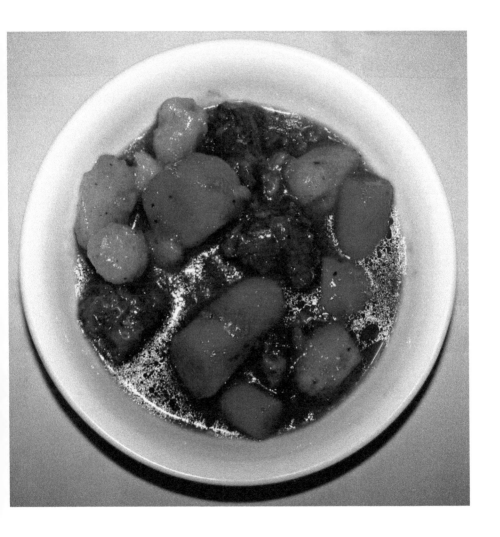

Bone Broth

Preparation time: 15 minutes

Cooking time: 6 hours

Servings: 8

Ingredients:

- 3 ½ lb. assorted mixed bones – ex. marrow bones, chicken feet, or your choice
- 1 tbsp. pink Himalayan salt

1 medium of each:

- Parsnip
- White onion – skin on
- 5 peeled garlic cloves
- 2 mediums of each:
- Celery stalks
- Carrots
- 2 tbsp. apple cider vinegar or lemon juice
- 8 cups of water

Directions:

1. Peel and slice the vegetables with roots into 1/3-inch pieces. Slice the onion in half. Chop the celery into thirds. Add the bay leaves into the slow cooker.

2. Toss in the chosen bones (can also be pork). Pour the water up to ¾ capacity—along with the juice/vinegar and bay leaves. Sprinkle with the salt.

3. Secure the lid. Choose either low for ten hours or high six hours. You can simmer up to 48 hours. Remove the bits of veggies using a strainer. Set the bones aside to chill. Shred the meat and use it as desired.

4. Refrigerate the broth overnight. Scrape away the tallow (greasy layer) if desired. Use within five days or freeze. You can also keep it in the canning jars for up to 45 days.

Nutrition:

- Calories: 72
- Fat: 6g
- Carbs: 0.7g
- Protein: 3.6g

Cabbage & Ground Beef Soup

Preparation time: 15 minutes

Cooking time: 3 hours

Servings: 4

Ingredients:

- 2 tbsp. olive oil

½ cup chopped of each:

- Shallots
- Onions
- 2 minced garlic cloves
- 2 lb. ground beef
- 1 tsp each of:
- Salt
- Pepper
- Dried parsley
- ½ tsp dried oregano
- 16oz. marinara sauce
- 2 cups of riced cauliflower – ½ head
- 5 cups of low-sodium beef broth
- 8 cup of sliced cabbage – 1 large

Directions:

1. In a skillet on the med-high heat setting, warm up the oil. When hot, stir in the garlic, shallots, and onions. Sauté until softened. Stir in the beef—cooking until pink is gone.

2. Toss in the seasonings and marinara sauce. Fold in the riced cauliflower and stir well. Pour the fixings into the slow cooker.

3. Empty in the beef broth and cabbage. Stir. Prepare to cook for six hours on low or three on the high setting. When done, have a seat and enjoy it.

Nutrition:

- Calories: 312
- Carbs: 9.8g
- Fat: 15.2g
- Protein: 31.1g

Cheesy Mexican Chicken Soup

Preparation time: 15 minutes

Cooking time: 4 hours

Servings: 6

Ingredients:

- 1 ½ lb. chicken thighs
- 15oz. chicken broth
- 15 ½oz. chunky salsa – ex. Tostitos
- 8oz. Pepper Jack/Monterey cheese

Directions:

1. Cut out any bones and remove the fat from the chicken. Arrange them in the slow cooker. Mix in the rest of the fixings. Set the cooker using the low setting for six to eight hours or three to four on the high setting.

2. When the time is up, remove and shred the chicken. Put it back in the cooker to mingle with the juices for a minute or so. Stir and serve right out of the slow cooker.

Nutrition:

- Calories: 400
- Carbs: 5.1g
- Fat: 22.8g

- Protein: 28g

Chicken & Bacon Chowder

Preparation time: 15 minutes

Cooking time: 8 hours

Servings: 8

Ingredients:

- 1 trimmed – sliced leek
- 6oz. sliced cremini mushrooms
- 1 finely chopped shallot
- 1 med. thinly sliced sweet onion
- 4 minced garlic cloves
- 4 tbsp. butter – divided
- 2 diced celery ribs
- 2 cups of chicken stock – divided
- 1 lb. chicken breasts
- 1 pkg. (8oz.) cream cheese
- 1 lb. bacon – crispy & crumbled
- 1 cup of heavy cream

1 tsp of each:

- Sea salt
- Dried thyme
- Black pepper
- Garlic powder

Directions:

1. Using the low setting for one hour, add the shallot, garlic, leek, mushrooms, celery, onions, one cup of the chicken stock, black pepper, sea salt, and two tablespoons butter to the slow cooker. Secure the lid.

2. In a skillet, sear the chicken breasts over the med-high setting on the stovetop using the rest of the butter. It should take approximately five minutes per side—making sure they are browned evenly. Set aside on a platter.

3. Deglaze the pan with the rest of the stock using a rubber spatula. Add the chicken to the slow cooker and pour in the cream, garlic powder, thyme, and cream cheese. Combine the mixture until the chunks of cheese are consumed in the mixture.

4. After the chicken has cooled down, cut it into cubes, and toss it into the cooker along with the bacon. Mix well. Cover and simmer for six to eight hours (low). When done, serve, and enjoy.

Nutrition:

- Calories: 355
- Carbs: 5.75g
- Fat: 28g
- Protein: 21g

Kale & Chicken Soup

Preparation time: 15 minutes

Cooking time: 6 hours

Servings : 6

Ingredients:

- 2lb. chicken thighs/breast meat
- 1/3 cup of onion
- ½ cup (+) 1 tbsp. olive oil
- 14oz. chicken broth
- 32oz. chicken stock
- 5oz. baby kale leaves
- Salt & pepper to taste
- ¼ cup of lemon juice

Also Needed:

- Large skillet
- Blender

Directions:

1. Remove all skin, including bones, from the chicken. Dice the onions. Heat-up one tbsp of the oil in a frying pan (med. heat). Sprinkle the pepper and salt on the chicken. Toss it into the pan.

2.   Lower the temperature to med-low and cover. Continue cooking the chicken until it reaches the internal temperature of 165°F (approximately 15 minutes).

3.   Shred your cooked chicken, and add it to the slow cooker. Use the blender to combine the rest of the oil, onion, and chicken broth.

4.   Scrape it into the cooker. Stir in the rest of the ingredients and cover. Prepare for 6 hours. Stir a few times during the final cycle. Serve and enjoy.

Nutrition:
- Calories: 261
- Carbs: 2g
- Protein: 14.1g
- Fat: 21g

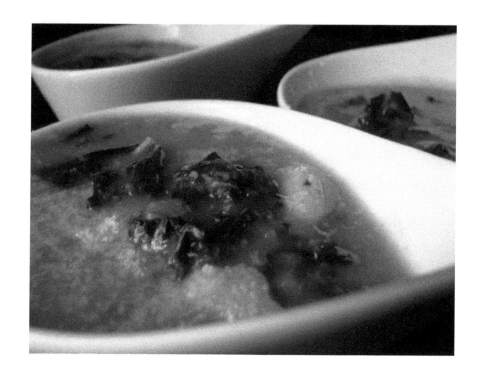

Reuben Soup with Thousand Island Dressing

Preparation time: 15 minutes

Cooking time: 8 hours

Servings: 12

Ingredients:

- 1 medium diced onion
- 8 cups of beef broth/stock
- 3 minced garlic cloves
- 2 tbsp. butter
- 2lbs. diced corned beef
- 1 lb. Sauerkraut
- 1 tbsp. mustard seeds

1 tsp of each:

- Dill seeds
- Coriander seeds

1 Hour Before Serving:

- 8oz. shredded Swiss cheese
- 2 cups of heavy cream

For the Topping:

- Thousand Island dressing

Directions:

1. Use the medium heat setting to brown the onion and garlic using one tablespoon of butter. Sauté for two minutes.

2. Stir in the beef broth, remaining butter, garlic, onions, mustard seeds, sauerkraut, corned beef, and beef broth. Prepare the soup using the high setting for 3.5 hours or 7 hours on low.

3. Approximately one hour before dinner, add the whipping cream and Swiss cheese. Top if off with the Thousand Island dressing as desired.

Nutrition:

- Calories: 343
- Carb: 1.3g
- Fat: 25.6g
- Protein: 22.8g

Sausage & Pepper Soup

Preparation time: 15 minutes

Cooking time: 5 hours

Servings: 4

Ingredients:

- 1 ½ lb. hot Italian sausage
- 2 cups of beef stock
- 6 cups of raw spinach
- ½ med. onion
- 1 medium of each: red & green bell pepper
- 1 can tomato with jalapenos
- ½ tsp kosher salt

2 tsp of each:

- Minced garlic
- Cumin
- Chili powder
- 1 tsp Italian seasoning

Directions:

1. Break the sausage into chunks and cook. Slice the green peppers. Toss the peppers, stock, and spices into the slow cooker. Arrange the sausage on top and mix well.

2. Fry the garlic and onions and add to the slow cooker. Toss the spinach and prepare using the high setting for three hours. Stir, and reduce the heat to the low setting for another two hours of cooking. Stir and serve.

Nutrition:

- Calories: 612.25
- Protein: 27.11g
- Carbs: 7.81g
- Fat: 50.79g

Spring Keto Stew with Venison

Preparation time: 20 minutes

Cooking Time: 6 hours

Servings: 2

Ingredients:

- 1lb. venison stew meat
- 1/2 cup purple cabbage, shredded
- 1/2 cup celery, sliced
- 2 cup bone broth

Directions:

1. Sauté cabbage and celery with olive oil and garlic in a skillet. Add the venison and season with salt and pepper to taste. Stir until meat is browned. Transfer everything into the crockpot. Add the cone broth. Cover and cook on low for 6 hours.

Nutrition:

- Calories: 310
- Fat: 16g

- Carbs: 5g
- Protein: 32g

Mexican Taco Soup

Preparation time: 5 minutes

Cooking Time: 4 hours

Servings: 2

Ingredients:

- 1lb. ground meat, browned
- 8oz cream cheese
- 10oz diced tomatoes and chilis
- 1 tbsp of taco seasonings
- 1 cup of chicken broth

Directions:

1. Combine all ingredients in the crockpot. Cook on low for 4 hours. Serve.

Nutrition:

- Calories: 547
- Fat: 43g
- Carbs: 5g
- Protein: 33g

Oxtail Stew

Preparation time: 20 minutes

Cooking Time: 10 hours

Servings: 2

Ingredients:

- 2lb. oxtail, chopped
- 10 tomatoes, diced
- 4 tsp paprika

Directions:

1. Place oxtail in the crockpot with water filling up to half the pot. Cover and cook for 10 hours on low. When cooked, transfer the oxtail to a saucepan and add the tomatoes paprika and other desired seasonings (garlic cloves, chili powder, salt). Stew for 15 minutes.

Nutrition:

- Calories: 456
- Fat: 29g
- Carbs: 7g

- Protein: 37g

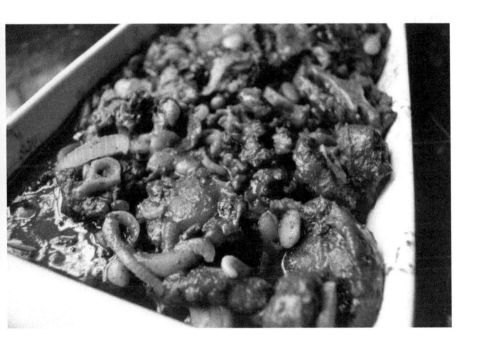

Rosemary Turkey and Kale Soup

Preparation time : 20 minutes

Cooking Time : 8 hours

Servings : 2

Ingredients:
- 2 carrots, sliced
- 2 cups turkey stock
- 1 sprig rosemary
- 2 cups turkey meat, bite-size pieces
- 2 cups kale, chopped

Directions:
1. Sauté onion, carrots, and desired spices in a skillet, then add half of the stock to deglaze. Put the turkey in the crockpot and add the contents of the skillet. Cover and cook for 8 hours on low. Add the kale when cooked.

Nutrition:
- Calories: 403
- Fat: 28g

- Carbs: 6g
- Protein: 34g

Onion Bison Soup

Preparation time: 50 minutes

Cooking Time: 6 hours

Servings: 2

Ingredients:

- 3 red onions, sliced 1/4-inch thick
- 1lb. bison roast
- 1 qt beef stock
- 1/4 cup sherry
- 2 sprigs thyme

Directions:

1. Place bison roast, stock, and thyme in the crockpot. Cover and cook on high within 6 hours. Sauté onions on a pot on medium heat.

2. Add sherry and cook for 3 minutes. Add the contents of the crockpot, seasoning with salt and pepper to taste. Let simmer for 45 minutes.

Nutrition:

- Calories: 517
- Fat: 30g
- Carbs: 7g
- Protein: 46g

Lamb Feet Stew

Preparation time: 30 minutes

Cooking Time: 10 hours

Servings: 2

Ingredients:

- 1 tsp coriander seeds
- 1 tsp black peppercorns
- 1 1/2lbs. lamb's feet
- 15oz peeled tomatoes
- 1/2 tsp each ground cayenne pepper and turmeric

Directions:

1. Broil the feet, 10 minutes on each side. Meanwhile, combine all ingredients in a food processor. Include onions, garlic, and ginger to taste.

2. Put the blended ingredients into a crockpot and add the broiled feet. Cover and cook for 10 hours on low.

Nutrition:

- Calories: 423
- Fat: 37g
- Carbs: 4g
- Protein: 35g

Curried Tomato Soup

Preparation time: 10 minutes

Cooking Time: 6 hours

Servings: 2

Ingredients:

- 2lb. ripe tomatoes, chopped
- 1 cup full-fat coconut milk
- 1 tsp curry powder

Directions:

1. Add all ingredients into the crockpot. Cook on low within 6 hours. Serve.

Nutrition:

- Calories: 306
- Fat: 17g
- Carbs: 2g
- Protein: 19g

Cream of Celery Soup

Preparation time: 10 minutes

Cooking Time: 6 hours

Servings: 2

Ingredients:

- 3 cups celery, diced
- 1/2 cup coconut milk
- 1 cup broth
- 1/2 teaspoon dill

Directions:

1. Add all ingredients into the crockpot. Add 1/2 onion and a pinch of salt. Cover and cook for 6 hours on low. When cooked, mix in an immersion blender.

Nutrition:

- Calories: 324
- Fat: 19g
- Carbs: 1g
- Protein: 17g

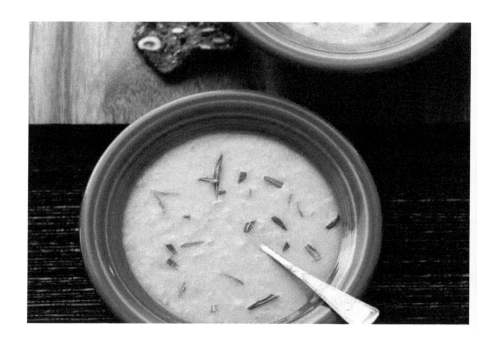

Tomato Basil Soup

Preparation time: 10 minutes

Cooking Time: 6 hours

Servings: 2

Ingredients:

- 30oz tomatoes, diced
- 6 large basil leaves
- 1/4 tbsp dried thyme
- 1/4 cup heavy cream
- 1/4 cup grated Parmesan cheese

Directions:

1. Except for the last two ingredients, combine all ingredients in an immersion blender with desired seasonings (onion, garlic, pepper, and spices) to taste. Transfer into the crockpot and cook on low for 6 hours. While hot, stir in heavy cream and Parmesan.

Nutrition:

- Calories: 294

- Fat: 14g
- Carbs: 2g
- Protein: 19g

Homemade Ketchup

Preparation time: 15 minutes

Cooking time: 7 hours

Servings: 2

Ingredients:

- 1 cup no-sugar tomato puree
- ¼ cup apple cider vinegar
- ¼ cup of water
- 3 drops of liquid stevia
- 1 small chopped onion
- 2 minced garlic cloves
- 2 tablespoons granulated stevia
- 1/8 teaspoon ground cloves
- 1/8 teaspoon ground allspice
- 1 teaspoon of sea salt
- Dash of black pepper

Directions:

1. Put all the listed fixing in your slow cooker and stir well. Cook on low for 6-7 hours. When time is up, puree the

ketchup, or blend in batches using a regular blender. Move ketchup to jars and cool to room temperature before sealing and storing in the fridge.

Nutrition:

- Calories: 19
- Protein: 1g
- Carbs: 4g
- Fat: 0g

Caramelized Onions

Preparation time: 15 minutes

Cooking time: 8 hours

Servings: 12

Ingredients:

- 4 big onions
- 4 tablespoons grass-fed butter
- ¼ cup balsamic vinegar

Directions:

1. Cut onions into slices about ¼-inch thick. Put in your slow cooker. Add butter and balsamic vinegar. Cook on low for 6-8 hours. Serve.

Nutrition:

- Calories: 72
- Protein: 1g
- Carbs: 6g
- Fat: 5g

Easy BBQ Sauce

Preparation time: 15 minutes

Cooking time: 8 hours

Servings: 4

Ingredients :

- 8-ounces canned no-sugar tomato sauce
- 2 tablespoons no-sugar Worcestershire sauce
- 2 tablespoons apple cider vinegar
- 2 tablespoons stone-ground mustard
- 1 tablespoon onion powder
- 1 tablespoon chili powder
- 2 teaspoons liquid smoke
- ¼ teaspoon garlic powder
- ½ teaspoon liquid stevia
- 1 teaspoon of sea salt
- Dash of black pepper

Directions:

1. Put all the listed fixing in your slow cooker. Cook on low within 6-8 hours. When time is up, use right away!

Nutrition:

- Calories: 56
- Protein: 1g
- Carbs: 11g
- Fat: 0g

Asian-Inspired BBQ Sauce

Preparation time: 15 minutes

Cooking time: 8 hours

Servings: 1

Ingredients:
- ¾ cup coconut aminos
- 6 tablespoons no-sugar tomato paste
- 6 tablespoons melted unsweetened almond butter
- 3 tablespoons apple cider vinegar
- 4 minced garlic cloves
- 3 teaspoons Dijon mustard
- 1 ½ teaspoons paprika
- Generous pinch of cinnamon
- Salt and pepper to taste

Directions:

1. Put all the fixing in your slow cooker. Cook on low for 6-8 hours. Use!

Nutrition:

- Calories: 105
- Protein: 3g
- Carbs: 9g
- Fat: 7g

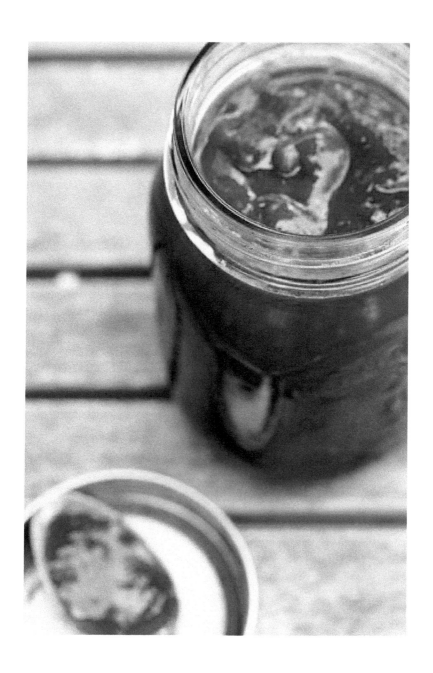

Alfredo Sauce

Preparation time: 15 minutes

Cooking time: 6 hours

Servings: 6

Ingredients:

- 3 ½ cups chicken broth
- 2 cups heavy cream
- 1 cup Parmesan cheese
- 5 minced garlic cloves
- ½ cup softened butter
- ¼ cup coconut flour
- 1 teaspoon dried parsley
- Salt and pepper to taste

Directions:

1. Grease your slow cooker with a coconut-oil based spray. Add chicken broth, cream, and garlic. Cook on low for 4-6 hours.

2. A half-hour before you plan to serve, mix butter, flour, and dried parsley in a bowl. Add to the slow cooker,

whisking until smooth. Cook until the sauce has thickened. Lastly, add in cheese to melt. Serve!

Nutrition:

- Calories: 255
- Protein: 4g
- Carbs: 3g
- Fat: 26g

Bacon-Whisky Jam

Preparation time: 15 minutes

Cooking time: 4 hours

Servings: 1

Ingredients:

- 14 slices bacon
- 1 cup black coffee
- 1 small chopped onion
- 7 drops liquid stevia
- 3 tablespoons apple cider vinegar
- 2 tablespoons granulated Sukrin Gold (brown sugar substitute)
- 1.5-ounces whisky
- 3 minced garlic cloves
- 1 tablespoon coconut aminos
- 1 tablespoon hot sauce
- 1 teaspoon no-sugar Worcestershire
- ¼ teaspoon pure maple extract
- Dash of black pepper

Directions:

1. Cook the bacon, then pat dry on a paper towel. Discard ½ of the fat from the skillet. Add garlic plus onion to the pan and cook in the remaining fat.

2. When nicely browned and fragrant, add in the rest of the ingredients. Bring to a boil, deglazing the pan by scraping up any stuck-on food bits.

3. Return bacon to the skillet. Pour the entire skillet into a slow cooker. Do not put on the lid, but cook uncovered for 3 ½ to 4 hours. Chop in a food processor before cooling. Serve.

Nutrition:
- Calories: 141
- Protein: 9g
- Carbs: 3g
- Fat: 7g

Green Tomato Chutney

Preparation time: 15 minutes

Cooking time: 8 hours

Servings: 2

Ingredients:

- 4 cups chopped green tomatoes
- ½ cup apple cider vinegar
- ¼ cup Red Boat fish sauce
- ¼ cup granulated erythritol
- 2 tablespoons chopped cilantro
- 2 tablespoons peeled and chopped ginger
- 2 tablespoons lime juice
- 2 chopped red chili peppers
- 1 tablespoon lime zest
- 1 teaspoon cinnamon
- 1 teaspoon salt
- 1 teaspoon onion powder
- ½ teaspoon ground allspice
- ½ teaspoon mustard powder
- ½ teaspoon ground cardamom
- ¼ teaspoon ground cloves

Directions:

1. Put everything in your slow cooker. Stir. Cook on high within 5 hours. When that time is up, stir, and cook again on low for 8-10 hours.

2. Spoon chutney into jars, leaving the liquid behind. Store in the fridge for up to 3 months (opened) or indefinitely (when unopened).

Nutrition:

- Calories: 40
- Protein: 3g
- Carbs: 6g
- Fat: 0g

Pumpkin Butter

Preparation time: 15 minutes

Cooking time: 5 hours

Servings: 9

Ingredients:

- 12 cups cooked pumpkin cubes
- ¼ cup apple cider vinegar
- 2 tablespoons Sukrin Gold (brown sugar substitute)
- 4 teaspoons ground cinnamon
- 2 teaspoons pure vanilla extract
- 2 teaspoons blackstrap molasses
- 2 teaspoons ground ginger
- 2 teaspoons salt
- ½ teaspoon nutmeg
- ½ teaspoon lucuma powder
- ¼ teaspoon granulated stevia

Directions:

1. Put all the fixing except apple cider vinegar and Sukrin Gold in the slow cooker. Cook on high within 2 hours, stirring every 40 minutes or so.

2. When time is up, blend with an immersion blender or in batches in a regular blender. Put back in the slow cooker. Whisk in vinegar and Sukrin Gold.

3. Taste, and add more seasonings if necessary. Close the lid, leaving it off-kilter a little, so there's a crack open, on high for 3 hours. Stir every hour.

4. When time is up, spoon into jars and cool before storing it in the fridge! Pumpkin butter should last unopened for a few months and opened for a few weeks.

Nutrition:

- Calories: 22
- Protein: 1g
- Carbs: 6g
- Fat: 0g

Pizza

Preparation time : 15 minutes

Cooking time: 6 hours

Servings: 8

Ingredients:

- 8 slices of pepperoni
- 1 lb. ground beef, cooked
- 1 cups spinach and your favorite pizza toppings
- 1 jar pizza sauce, unsweetened
- 2 cups shredded mozzarella cheese

Directions:

1. Combine the ground beef and pizza sauce in a bowl, and spread this mixture on the bottom of a 4-quart slow-cooker.

2. Top with the spinach leaves, and then with 8 pepperoni slices. Add your favorite toppings, such as sliced mushrooms, chopped green bell pepper, diced tomatoes, and minced garlic.

3. Cover with the mozzarella cheese, then seal the slow-cooker with its lid. Set the cooking timer for 4 to 6 hours and cook at a low heat setting. Allow the pizza cool slightly before slicing to serve.

Nutrition:

- Calories: 487
- Carbohydrates: 7.6g
- Fats: 37g
- Protein: 30g

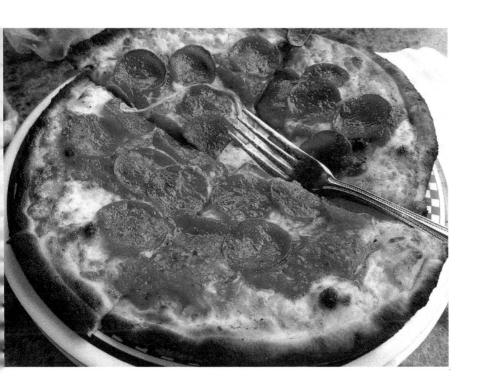

Cheese Artichoke Dip

Preparation time: 15 minutes

Cooking time: 3 hours

Servings: 8

Ingredients:

- 14oz. artichoke hearts, drained and chopped
- 1 red bell pepper, diced
- 16oz. grated mozzarella cheese
- 1 cup grated parmesan cheese
- 1 cup mayonnaise

Directions:

1. Place all the fixing apart from the cheese in a 4-quart slow-cooker, and stir until mixed. Cook on your slow cooker within 3 hours over the low setting.

2. Gently stir in the cheese, and continue cooking for an additional hour. Allow cooling before serving.

Nutrition:

- Calories: 386
- Carbohydrates: 8.9g
- Fats: 29g
- Protein: 2.1g

Cajun Chicken Stuffed Avocado

Preparation time: 15 minutes

Cooking time: 8 hours

Servings: 3

Ingredients:

- 3 avocados, stone removed and halved
- 3 chicken thighs
- 2 teaspoons Cajun seasoning
- 1/4 cup mayonnaise
- 2 tablespoons sour cream
- 2 tablespoons lemon juice

Directions:

1. Place the chicken into a 4-quart slow-cooker, sprinkle with the Cajun seasoning, and pour in 2 cups water. Cook within 8 hours, allowing it to cook at a low heat setting.

2. Remove the chicken, and shred it, using forks, and discarding the bones. Flavor the chicken with salt and cayenne pepper, add the remaining ingredients, apart from the avocado, and stir until well-combined.

3. Chop up half of each avocado into small pieces, and stir into the chicken mixture. Fill each remaining avocado half with the prepared chicken mixture. Serve a stuffed avocado half to each person, with some chicken and avocado salad alongside.

Nutrition:

- Calories: 638
- Carbohydrates: 21g
- Fats: 50.6g
- Protein: 34.5g

Parmesan Chicken Wings

Preparation time: 15 minutes

Cooking time: 3 hours

Servings: 4

Ingredients:

- 24 chicken wings
- 4 teaspoons minced garlic
- 1 tablespoon dried parsley
- 2 cups grated Parmesan cheese

Directions:

1. Place the chicken wings in a 4-quart slow-cooker. Place 1 cup of parmesan cheese, the garlic, and parsley in a separate bowl, mixing well. Season with salt and black pepper, then pour onto the chicken wings, tossing the wings to coat them well.

2. Cover and seal slow-cooker with its lid, then adjust the cooking timer for 2 ½ to 3 hours, allowing to cook at a high heat setting. In the meantime, switch on the grill and allow it to heat.

3. Transfer the chicken onto a large baking sheet, lined with a parchment sheet, and sprinkle with the remaining cheese.

4. Place the baking sheet under the grill, and allow to grill for 5 minutes, or until cheese has completely melted and the chicken wings are crispy. Serve immediately.

Nutrition:

- Calories: 223
- Carbohydrates: 0.8g
- Fats: 21.7g
- Protein: 25.1g

Tomato and Feta Cheese Dip

Preparation time: 15 minutes

Cooking time : 3 hours & 10 minutes

Servings: 8

Ingredients:

- 1 can tomatoes
- 1/2 white onion, peeled and diced
- 2 1/2 cups mixed basil, oregano, and parsley leaves
- 1/4 cup red wine
- 8oz. cubed feta cheese

Directions:

1. Put a medium-sized skillet over medium heat, add 2 tablespoons oil and allow to heat. Add the onion, and allow to cook for 5 to 7 minutes until the onion is soft.

2. Stir in 1 teaspoon of minced garlic and a pinch of crushed red pepper. Continue to cook for another 2 minutes, then add the wine.

3. Stir continuously until the wine evaporates, then stir in the herbs and tomatoes. Transfer this mixture into a 4-

quart slow-cooker, add the cheese, and season with salt and ground black pepper.

4. Cover and seal the slow-cooker with its lid, adjust the cooking timer for 3 hours, and cook at a high heat setting. Allow cooling before serving.

Nutrition:

- Calories: 182
- Carbohydrates: 7g
- Fats: 10g
- Protein: 4g

Chocolate Fondue

Preparation time: 15 minutes

Cooking time: 2 hours

Servings: 8

Ingredients:

- 2 1/2oz chopped chocolate, chopped and unsweetened
- 1/3 cup Swerve Sweetener, powdered
- 1/2 teaspoon vanilla extract, unsweetened
- 1 cup full-fat coconut cream

Directions:

1. Grease a 4-quart slow-cooker with a non-stick cooking spray and add all ingredients to it. Stir until combined, then cover and seal slow-cooker with its lid.

2. Adjust the cooking timer for 2 hours and allow to cook at a low heat setting until smooth. Serve as a dip with mixed fruit.

Nutrition:

- Calories: 154
- Carbohydrates: 3.7g
- Fats: 14.87g
- Protein: 1.8g

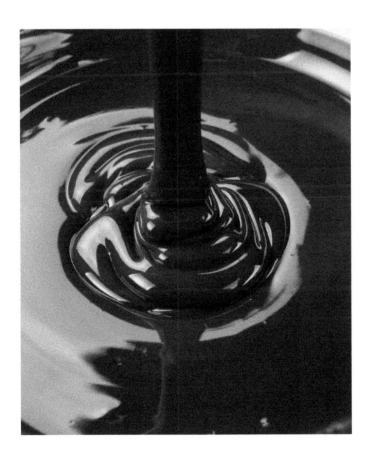

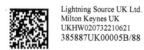

Lightning Source UK Ltd.
Milton Keynes UK
UKHW020732210621
385887UK00005B/88